Family And Alcoholism

The effects of alcoholism on spouses, children, and families

By

Nancy C. Davidson

Table of contents

Introduction

Do you occasionally indulge in a drink?Many of us do, frequently while interacting with friends and family.Depending on your age, health status, and, naturally, how much you drink, drinking can be beneficial or harmful.

Alcoholism is a disease that cannot be explained in simple terms.

In general, the condition of obsessive drinking despite health risks is known as alcohol addiction.Even though you are well aware of the harmful effects, alcoholism means that you have no control over your consumption.

An alcoholic drinks even if he gets into alcohol-related problems like drinking and driving and losing his job.

A person who drinks is not always an alcoholic.A person is not considered to be alcohol-dependent if he or she consumes alcohol in controlled amounts and is able to refuse when he or she does not want to.He or she simply drinks with friends.

This book contains useful information based on research for anyone who drinks.Consider your drinking habits and how they might affect your health. What do you think?You can use this as a starting point.

Chapter 1

The potency of booze: human inability to control demand

A lot of research was done to figure out what stops people from having happy and healthy lives.Drugs, money ,and unemployment each has its own value and impact.The fact that alcohol, but not other illicit drugs, posed a real threat to human life was not defined by government officials.It is critical to pay more attention to alcohol and its spread if we are to improve living conditions and comprehend the threat posed by alcohol.People are free to use any form of beauty because there are so many fascinating aspects to human existence.Nevertheless, individuals select the worst and most perilous ideas without taking into account the potential harm they could cause to themselves.

One of the most dangerous drinks available to people is alcohol.In order to take advantage of the alcoholic state, the vast majority of citizens of any nation are eager to spend money and neglect their health.So, why do so many people prefer to consume alcohol?In student hostels, one of the early stages when people decide to drink is observed.Young people often get the chance to live far from their parents and do whatever interests them.John Smith, a resident of the British hostel, admits that he first tried alcohol in his freshman year of college.Although there were no particular motivations for getting drunk, there was a desire to "taste an adult independent life."

When young students who are unable to clearly define the priorities of college life choose to try something bad that is still available rather than wait for something better that is not available right now, they make numerous mistakes.Although they can make quick decisions, students are still unable to arrive at some reasonable solutions.For instance, student prefer to attend nightclubs or parties where the effects of alcohol encourage communication and freedom in order to make new friends and enjoy college life.

John stated, "In fact, it was difficult to understand when it was better to stop; as a result, all students decided to drink as long as the opportunities permitted."The initial alcohol experience does not go as planned:The consequences of drinking bother some students.Because they can only be observed in the morning, the outcomes are probably one of the aspects of alcohol use that is the most unpredictable:terrible headache, giddiness, the need to remember what happened yesterday because you can't see where you are or what you're doing here, and the desire to drink again because the hangover is so strong.

Even though John's first alcohol experience was unsuccessful, it was not enough to convince him of the terrible effects of drinking.The primary threat is this:People don't think it's necessary to stop drinking because alcohol doesn't appear to be harmful.John concurs that the majority of his friends enjoy drinking just to socialize, spend time together, and benefit from the opportunities for communication.He explains that alcohol parties, when the boundaries between what is permissible and what is not, allowed him to meet his friends Many adults and students truly believe that drinking beer, Cafe Royal, or other low-alcohol beverages causes less harm.This choice is dangerous and incorrect.Vodka, brandy, and beer drinkers suffer the same consequences and become dependent on alcohol.The evaluation of whether drinking is necessary and the possible volume of the beverage is the actual decision that needs to be made.

Today, John thinks it's appropriate to drink beer to unwind, enjoy company, and be in good spirits.Naturally, there are times when consuming alcohol is necessary to reduce pain, forget something or someone, or prevent oneself from engaging in more harmful behavior, as John explains.A devastating loss took place in the life of one of John's friends.He lost a close relative to cancer that could no longer be treated.

The only option was to wait and believe, and there were no chances to save his life.He had to be tough and confident in every word he said, which was very important.Still, it was so difficult to deal with pain that satisfied the mind and body.His friend was able to forget about the danger, believe that good could happen, and assist other family members in becoming stronger as a result of a portion of the drinks.John believes that it is better to get drunk than to cry and curse everything, including In order to address the issues posed by alcohol, it is necessary to get the attention of the government and convince each representative of the potential dangers posed by alcohol.It will only be possible to inform citizens about the dangers posed by alcohol and the overwhelming majority of people's blind alcoholic dependence if the government takes some action. Alcohol comes in many forms, and most people have no idea how they can become dependent on it.The fact that individuals themselves produce alcohol to make themselves dependent, less secure, and weak in the face of truth and dependence is a form of evil fate.

Chapter 2

Alternative Approaches to Alcoholism Treatment

In recent years, alternative methods of treating alcoholism have gained popularity.This method of treatment incorporates both conventional and cutting-edge scientific approaches to the treatment of particular symptoms.

Alcoholism requires a different approach to treatment than other diseases.It is necessary to make an effort to create environments that are stress-free.

Different rehab centers around the world offer treatment that addresses the person's entire life, not just their symptoms.

This necessitates locating and eliminating the root causes of the dependency.

In healing sessions at detox centers, patients are gently guided to open their deepest concerns and fears.This helps identify the habit's underlying cause.

After that, a positive treatment plan is created to help the patient break his habit and continue living a happy and healthy life.

Clinical depression may contribute to alcoholism.In these instances, treatment necessitates more in-depth mental preparation.These individuals are enrolled in psychotherapeutic treatment programs, which are an effective alternative treatment for this condition.The patient's emotional and addictive layers are both addressed by this treatment.

Religious counseling is also becoming more popular as a treatment option for alcoholism.A person's spiritual beliefs may be a major factor in his decision to stop drinking.

Addicts can learn a variety of meditation techniques from spiritual leaders from a variety of organizations. These techniques help addicts overcome stress and find peace, making it easier for them to kick their habit and start living a calm and peaceful life.

Yoga, various forms of meditation, and trance are all methods. A person can relax his or her mind and become stress-free and unaffected by meditation if they focus on themselves.

When a person is happy and content with himself, he is unaffected by what is going on around him and no longer needs anything that makes him feel happy, at ease, and peaceful.

Because they believe that meditation is superior to medication, many people enroll in this kind of program.Meditating provides one with a solution that lasts, whereas medicine is temporary.

Trance work is similar to meditation in some ways.This provides the addict with tremendous inner strength to assist him in mastering his enticements with relative ease and helps the individual center his mind on studying deeper truths.

Yoga which is really famous now is an alternate viable treatment

methodology for the state of liquor abuse.Yoga alleviates anxiety and helps a person effectively reduce stress and tension.Yoga promotes effective harmony between the body and the brain through gentle stretching.

Nutritional counseling is a different type of alternative treatment that has been shown to be effective.

Excessive alcohol consumption is the cause of numerous nutritional deficiencies,Because the alcoholic's small intestine is no longer capable of absorbing essential nutrients, his body stops absorbing them, which contributes to his health.

After quitting drinking, nutritional counseling may be of assistance.

In most cases, he or she receives a counseling evaluation and is given a diet plan to follow in order to return to a healthy and active lifestyle.This includes bringing the blood sugar level of the recovering individual back into balance.

Acupuncture is one more effective alternative treatment.In a number of cases, this has been successful.Patients are instructed by acupuncturists to use this as a complement to other treatments.

Chapter 3

Alcoholism in Relationships

In the United States, married couples frequently consume alcohol.About half of all couples have husbands and wives who drink alcohol frequently (at once a month or more).

Only a quarter of all couples do not drink on a regular basis, and another quarter of those surveyed have a husband who does not drink on a regular basis but the wife does.Only 5% of married couples in the United States have a wife who drinks regularly and a husband who does not. This is a significant example of gender differences.

Married couples have a lower prevalence of heavy alcohol consumption—defined as 14 or more drinks per week for men and 10 or more for women.In 4% of married couples, neither partner is a heavy drinker, and in 79%, neither partner is a heavy drinker.Again, there are differences between the sexes, with 12% of couples having only a heavy drinker husband and 5% having only a heavy drinker wife.

What are the repercussions?

People can frequently consume moderate amounts of alcohol with relatively few side effects.However, excessive alcohol consumption can have numerous negative effects on marriage.

Lower marital satisfaction is linked to heavy drinking, alcoholism, and alcohol use disorders.When the husband is the problem drinker, this connection is a little stronger, but it still holds true when the wife is the problem drinker.

Physical and psychological alcohol use is a factor in domestic violence and aggression, whether committed by the perpetrator or the victim.

Alcohol and substance abuse are among the most common causes of divorce, coming in at number three for women and number eight for men.Additionally, it is one of the most frequently cited reasons for seeking marriage counseling.

Compared to couples in which neither partner has an alcohol use disorder, couples in which one partner has an alcohol use disorder (usually alcohol dependence) have more negative interactions and fewer positive interactions.

A couple's content can be entirely different depending on how much they drink.

The negative effects of excessive alcohol consumption can be at their most severe when there is a significant disparity in the amount of alcohol consumed by each spouse.On the other hand, some studies have shown that couples who drink similar amounts together may not experience as many negative effects.The results show:

Marital satisfaction is higher in couples where both partners drink heavily than in couples where one partner only drinks heavily.

Compared to couples in which only one partner has an alcohol use disorder, couples in which both spouses have an alcohol use disorder have a greater number of positive interactions and a greater proportion of positive interactions to negative interactions.

Divorce rates are lower in couples in which both partners regularly consume alcohol than in those in which one partner does not.

All things considered, couples in which the two life partners drink vigorously might be bound to drink all together action, subsequently representing more sure communications.Indeed, couples who consume similar amounts of alcohol but do not drink together do not enjoy the same relationship benefits as couples who do.

But how about the youngsters?

It is essential to keep in mind that these findings speak to the effects of alcohol consumption on marriage.Even though couples who drink heavily together have fewer issues in their relationships than couples in which only one partner drinks heavily, the outcomes for their children are different.When both parents are heavy drinkers, children have worse outcomes than when only one parent is.

Couples in which both partners drink a lot may have a higher rate of physical aggression, which can hurt children.Couples report the most husband-perpetrated physical aggression when both partners consume a lot of alcohol or are more dependent on alcohol.When one spouse is more dependent, wife-perpetrated physical aggression occurs more frequently and does not decrease when both spouses are dependent.

Chapter 4

Are you ready to quit

Are you willing to modify your drinking habits?

How many times have you told yourself, "I need to stop drinking alcohol, I can't take this any longer"?Assuming you're dependent on liquor you've probably expressed this to yourself and conceivably others more times than you can count.The question is, are you actually prepared to stop?

Know where you are in the process and what to do. The problem is that the part of you that is addicted won't join the part of you that wants to stop and that will be your first obstacle to quitting drinking.Your dependent side will never want to stop drinking.

The healthy part of you is aware of the harm that alcohol is doing to you and that this situation has gone way over the top; however, the dependent part of you will never want to stop drinking for good.

If you can even conceive of a life without alcohol, it would be too horrible.And it's a scary step into the strange to walk away from something that has become such an integral part of your life with predictable (on some level, consoling) outcomes.

First and foremost, you must evaluate your circumstances.You need to be completely open with yourself and examine the negative effects that alcohol has had on your life in detail.And be aware that if you continue to drink, your life will continue to deteriorate.

Your life might look good from the outside for some of the more active drinkers.But people who seem to be "pulling it off" are more likely to end up with serious health problems or even die from common drinking illnesses like cirrhosis because they don't feel the urge to stop drinking as soon as someone who has been "knocked down" by alcohol earlier in their drinking.

This kind of drinker experiences a variety of effects much earlier than the functional drinker does, and as a result, they are more likely to seek assistance sooner.

If drinking is putting a lot of stress on you, and you've decided that you've had enough of the ongoing problems that alcohol addiction causes, you'll need to be brave enough to start. You'll also need to choose a good plan in the form of help to stop drinking on a regular basis, which will take away everything you care about from your life.

You'll need to decide whether to cut back or stop drinking if you want to change your drinking habits.

It's a good idea to talk about different options with a doctor, a friend, or someone else you trust.

If any of the following applies to you:

If none of the above applies to you, then talk to your doctor about whether you should cut back or quit based on factors like:

'Family history of alcohol issues' 'Your age' 'Whether you've had wounds related to drinking' 'Symptoms like sleep disorders and sexual dysfunction' 'If you choose to cut back or stop, and make a change plan.

If you continue to have mixed feelings, don't be surprised.Before you feel confident in your decision, you may need to reconsider it multiple times.

Even if you have committed yourself to making a change, you may occasionally experience mixed emotions.Creating a written "change plan" will help you set goals, explain why you want to reach them, and figure out how to get there.

This page contains a sample form.

Goal: (select one) I would like to consume no more than _____ on any given day and no more than _____ per week.

I would like to stop drinking.

Timing:

I will begin at this time:

Reasons:

These changes are necessary for me for the following reasons:

Consider the following alternatives in the interim if you believe you are not yet ready to take any action:

Keep track of how much and how often you drink, as well as how it affects you. Make a list of the benefits and drawbacks of changing your behavior. Deal with other priorities that might get in the way. Ask for help from your doctor, a friend, or someone you trust. Consider taking precautions.

Chapter 5

Handling Urges

The advice that follows will give you ideas to help you decide to cut back or stop drinking.They are not intended to replace professional assistance and can be used in conjunction with counseling or therapy.If you decide to try them on your own and find that you need more help at any point, get help.

Manage your drinking urges with a little help As you change your drinking habits, it's normal to have cravings or urges to drink.The terms "urge" and "craving" refer to a wide range of thoughts, bodily sensations, or emotions that make you want to drink despite your strong desire not to.

You might sense a loss of control or be uncomfortable being pulled in two directions.

Luck has it that drinking urges are fleeting, predictable, and manageable.In this section, we present a recognize-avoid-cope strategy, which is commonly used in cognitive behavioral therapy to assist individuals in changing unhelpful thought processes and behaviors.

You will find that your urges to drink will become less powerful over time as you use new responses, and you will gain confidence in your ability to deal with urges that may still occur from time to time.

Consult a doctor or therapist for support if you're having a really hard time with urges or if you don't make any progress with these techniques after a few weeks.Additionally, it may be easier to stop drinking with some new, non-habit-forming medications that can lessen or eliminate the urge to drink.

Recognize two types of "triggers": external stimuli in one's environment and internal stimuli within oneself can both trigger an urge to drink.

a. People, places, things, or times of day that offer drinking opportunities or encourage you to drink are known as "external triggers."In contrast to internal triggers, these "risky situations" are more obvious, predictable, and avoidable.

b. As the urge to drink appears to "pop up," internal triggers may be puzzling.But if you don't think about it when it happens, you might find that the urge was caused by a fleeting thought, a positive or negative emotion like excitement or frustration, or a physical sensation like a headache, tension, or nervousness. Consider keeping track of your urges to drink and examining them for a few weeks.This will assist you with getting more mindful of when and how you go through urges, what sparkles them, and ways of forestalling or controlling them.

Avoid risky situations In most cases, your best strategy will be to avoid taking the chance that you will act on your impulse and then drink.Drink little or no alcohol at home.Avoid social activities that involve drinking.If declining an invitation

makes you feel self-conscious, remind yourself that you are not necessarily saying "forever."
You might decide to gradually ease into a few situations that you have now decided to avoid if the urges lessen or become more manageable.
In the meantime, you can keep in touch with your friends by suggesting other activities that don't involve drinking.

You will need a variety of strategies to address impulses to drink because it is impossible to avoid all risky situations or to block internal triggers.
Some options are as follows:

- Prompt yourself of your justification for rolling out an improvement.Keep your top reasons on a wallet card or in an electronic message that you can easily access, such as a saved email or a notepad entry on your phone.

- Discuss it with someone you can rely on.Keep a trusted acquaintance on call in case of an emergency, or bring one with you to potentially dangerous situations.

- Find a new activity to keep you occupied.Choose engaging short, mid-range, and long options for various situations, such as texting or calling someone, watching a short video on the internet, lifting weights to music, taking a shower, meditating, going for a walk, or engaging in a leisure activity.

- Disagree with the thought that inspires the urge.Stop it,
concentrate on the issue in it, and substitute it.An illustration:It wouldn't hurt to drink a little.Please pause for a moment—what am I thinking?As I have witnessed, "simply one" can result in many more.I'm going to stick to my decision not to drink."

- Keep going through it without giving way.Accept an urge as normal and fleeting rather than fighting it.Keep in mind that it will soon peak and vanish like an ocean wave as you ride it out.

- Disappear gracefully and quickly from risky situations.Planning your escape in advance helps.

Chapter 6

Personal Connection to Alcohol Abuse

Given that alcohol abuse affects numerous families, ruins people's health, and harms their social lives.A variety of acute and chronic diseases are brought on by alcohol use disorder, which is probably the most preventable cause of death.For instance, it is undeniable that excessive alcohol consumption may result in esophageal cancer, pancreatitis, hypertension, gastric ulcers, liver cirrhosis, neurologic and psychiatric disorders, and hypertension.In order to assist patients in overcoming addiction and preventing long-term health consequences, substance use disorder sometimes necessitates institutionalization and prolonged treatment.Consequently, screening's early detection of the issue and prompt intervention are considered crucial.However, many addicts refuse to acknowledge the difficulties they face when they consume alcohol.Since I was a child, I've been afraid of spirits because I've seen how bad alcoholism can make people.It is important to note that counseling is an important part of helping people who abuse alcohol;It is crucial in bringing addicts back to a healthy life and ending this fatal addiction.

Addiction to alcohol is tragic for addicts and their families, and counseling may not be effective in changing an addict's attitude and behavior toward alcohol and preventing relapse.When I was 16 years old, my uncle passed away at the age of 50 from stage four hepatocellular carcinoma.Because the cancer had spread to other organs at that point, chemotherapy only extended his life by one year.He drank a lot for a long time, which caused him to lose his job, get divorced, have a lot of debt, and die from a terminal illness.My uncle's addiction was known to everyone in our family, but he refused to admit it and refused counseling.He took part in cognitive behavioral therapy, which should assist people in overcoming alcohol-related attitude disorders.My uncle, who was not yet ready to admit his addiction, was not helped by this strategy, which calls for a discussion about the patient's emotions.The main problem in my uncle's case was that it affected his health as well as his social status.I witnessed my well-educated uncle's insane behavior when he was drunk because he lived with us for two years.As a result, I was reluctant to try alcohol until recently and thought it was unacceptable .

Additionally, hearing about my uncle's story made me acutely aware of other people's substance abuse issues.

In conclusion, alcohol abuse is a serious health and social issue that can lead to a variety of acute and chronic illnesses, as well as social withdrawal, which makes intervention and recovery more difficult.The story of my uncle shows how a person's life and health can be destroyed by alcoholism and refusing counseling.contrary to that.Because of these incident involving member of my family, I became more aware of other people's substance abuse issues.As a result, I frequently request regular screening for alcohol abuse and other health issues from friends who drink.

Chapter 7

Saying No Skill

"Social pressure" to drink from acquaintances or other people may make it difficult to cut back or stop, even if you are committed to changing your drinking habits.This chapter offers a recognize-avoid-cope strategy, which is used in cognitive-behavioral therapy to help people change their negative thinking and behavior.

Turn It Down Recognize Two Types of Pressure The first step is to become aware of the Direct and Indirect Types of Social Pressure to Drink Alcohol.

If you are offered a drink or the opportunity to drink, you are subject to direct social pressure.

Even if no one offers you a drink, indirect social pressure is when you feel compelled to drink just by being around other people who are drinking.

Consider the circumstances in which you are subjected to direct or indirect pressure to drink excessively.You can record them in writing.Then, for each circumstance, select one or more resistance strategies from the list below or develop your own.

It's important to avoid pressure whenever possible. For some situations, your best strategy may be to avoid them all together.Remind yourself that you are not necessarily saying "eternally" if you find yourself feeling guilty about postponing an event or declining an invitation.

When you have self-assurance in your resistance abilities, you might decide to gradually enter situations you are now avoiding.In the meantime, you can keep in touch with friends by suggesting other things to do that don't involve drinking.

Recognize your "no" When you know alcohol will be served, it is essential to prepare a few resistance strategies in advance. Face situations you can't avoidYou'll need to be prepared to say a convincing "no thanks" if you want to be offered a drink.Your objective should be straightforward, steadfast, and friendly at the same time.Avoid lengthy explanations and weak justifications because they tend to prolong the discussion and give you more reason to give in.

Several additional considerations should be made:

Keep your response brief, clear, and concise. The person offering you a drink may not be aware that you are attempting to cut back or quit, and their level of consistency may vary. "Don't waver, as that will give you the opportunity to dream up reasons to go along "If the individual persists, it's a good idea to plan a series of responses, from a straightforward refusal to a more assertive response.

Think about the following sequence:

No, thank you.

"No, I don't want to, thank you.

"You know, I'm cutting back on alcohol now to get in shape, take care of myself, and do what my doctor told me to do."If you could assist me, I would truly appreciate it.

Additionally, you can try the "broken record" method.You simply need to repeat the same concise response each time the individual makes a statement.You might want to acknowledge a portion of the people's points (like, "I hear you...") before returning to your off-the-record response (like, "...but no thank you").And you can walk away if your words fail.

Script and practice your "no"

A ton of people are flabbergasted at how hard it very well might be to say no the

first two or multiple times.By writing out your lines and practicing them, you can boost your confidence.First things first, picture the situation and the person holding the drink.Then, write what the person will say and how you'll respond, whether it's a broken record strategy like the one described above or your own unique strategy.

To become more comfortable with your delivery and choice of words, say it out loud.In a similar vein, you might want to consider asking someone who is there for you to role play with you. This person might put you under honest pressure to drink and give you honest feedback on your answers.You will learn as you go, whether you practice through fictitious or real-life experiences.

If you keep at it, your tools will get better over time.

Try other strategies In addition to being fixed with your "no thank you," consider the following strategies:

Keep a record of each drink if you're cutting down so you stay within your limits. Invite support from other people to fight temptation. Plan an escape if the enticement gets too big. Ask other people to refrain from pressuring you or drinking in your presence (this may be difficult). If you've successfully declined drink offers in the past, remember what worked and build on it.

Keep in mind that you have a choice. Your success may be affected by how you decide to change your habits.A lot of people who decide to cut back on or stop drinking think, "I'm not allowed to drink," as though rules are being enforced by someone else.These kinds of thoughts may lead to resentment and make it simpler to give in.This way of thinking must be challenged by telling yourself that you are in control, that you know how you want your life to be, and that you have chosen to change.

In a similar vein, if you make a change, you might be concerned about how others will perceive you or react to you.Again, challenge these ideas by remembering that this is your life, that you have the choice, and that your decision should be respected.

Chapter 8

What is the most effective strategy for confronting an alcoholic regarding their drinking problem?

Please be aware that confronting an alcoholic will rarely result in a positive outcome.They are much more likely to continue drinking and feel the need to justify their actions.

The majority of families may find that staging an intervention improves their chances.A trained interventionist is the only person who should carry out this.They are well-versed in what to say and how to direct the family through the entire process.

Interventions frequently result in the alcoholic's consent to seek addiction treatment.Because it works well most of the time, it should be considered by more families.

Conclusion

This can be a difficult journey, and you might make mistakes along the way...

Get back on track right away.Stop drinking as soon as possible.

Keep in mind that each day is a new start.You don't have to keep drinking, even if you slip, which can be frightening.

You are in charge of making your choices.

Recognize that failures are common when making significant changes.Your long-term progress is what matters.

"Don't beat yourself up."It is of no use.You should never let feelings of disappointment, resentment, or guilt prevent you from seeking assistance and getting back on track.

Seek assistance.Talk about what happened right away with your counselor or a sober friend who supports you, or go to an AA or other mutual-help meeting.

Thoroughly consider it.Work on your own or with assistance to better comprehend why the incident occurred at that specific time and location with a limited amount of space.

"Learn from what happened."Write down what you need to do to prevent it from happening again.Make the most of the experience to strengthen your commitment.

Avoid situations that encourage drinking.Eliminate alcohol from your home.Avoid reliving the circumstances in which you drank, if at all possible.

Find alternate options.Keep busy with things that have nothing to do with drinking.

Best of luck with your project.

www.ingramcontent.com/pod-product-compliance
Lightning Source LLC
Chambersburg PA
CBHW071245140726
47996CB00007B/2764